So, You're Getting Chemo...

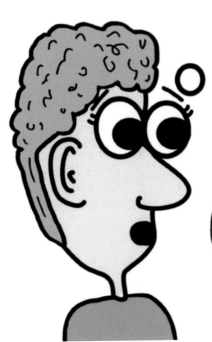

A funny guide for adult cancer patients in chemotherapy.

Tracy Wazac

This book is dedicated to:

My husband, Michael, for being my rock while I was going through hell.

My mom, for being there when I needed you the most.

The medical staff at The Holden Comprehensive Cancer Center at the University of Iowa Hospitals and Clinics for saving my life.

All of the people who are fighting cancer and who have fought it in the past.

What this book is:

Funny

Relatable

Full of cuss words

Blunt

Something to put you in a positive frame of mind while you (or a loved one) is attempting to kick cancer's ass

What this book isn't:

Sappy

For kids or people easily offended

Inspirational

Written by a doctor

Long story short, you are in a shitty situation right now. Chemo sucks. This book will hopefully show you that you are not alone and that it is okay to laugh about certain aspects of your life right now. This book is written by a chemo survivor who is not a doctor. Please consult your physician before taking any of this advice.

Cancer Can Eat a Bag of Dicks

Throughout this book, I am providing tips. You can find them in little boxes.

Just remember that this is what worked for me, so if my unsolicited advice isn't your cup of tea, don't get all offended.

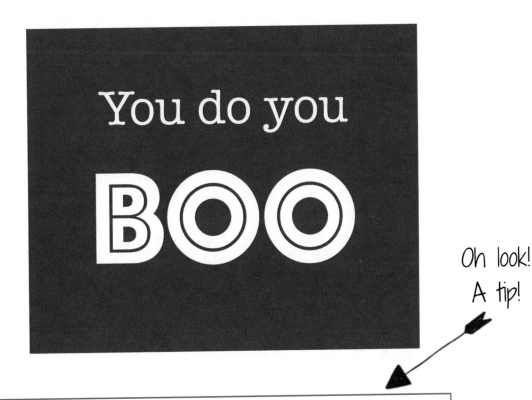

You do you

BOO

Oh look!
A tip!

Tip: As much as it sucks and as shitty as you look, take pictures. It is surreal looking back. Who knows, you might write a book someday.

I wish cancer would get cancer and die.

Been There, Done That

Hi, my name is Tracy and I put together this book because I know first hand what you are experiencing. A few years ago, I was diagnosed with breast cancer and it wasn't the "easy" kind. Mine was triple negative and because it was aggressive, I got to have chemo. Good times...

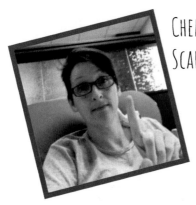

Chemo 1
Scared as hell.

Chemo 3
So over
this shit.

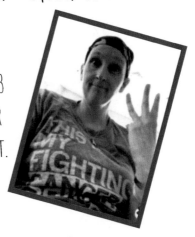

Chemo does weird shit to you. Everyone knows you are probably going to lose your hair and get sick, but there are so many more side effects that you will probably experience. There is stuff that they don't tell you or that is more anecdotal. I'm using this book as an opportunity to "warn" you, with humor.

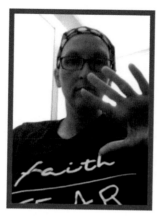

Chemo 5
Giving zero fucks
(I actually vomited during this one)

Laughter got me through most days and there were other days when I would just cry. Cancer is scary because you are literally facing the possibility that you could die. And if you make it through, you will never be the same person that you were before. Welcome to the club that you never wanted to join.

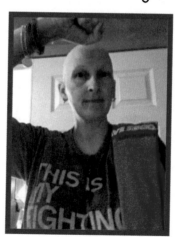

Chemo 8
My last one. I took all of the wearable gifts from friends. The support was amazing.

Since I'm writing and making doodles to create this book, I obviously got through it. I had 8 rounds of dose dense chemo. I had the steroids and the anti nausea meds (multiple kinds because I was a puker). I lost my hair. I couldn't poop. I gained about 20 pounds. My fingernails turned brown and my right foot was numb. My hair went from brown and curly to straight and gray. My eyesight was permanently affected and I think that my front two teeth are a slightly different color.

My bald husband shaving my head. I looked terrified.

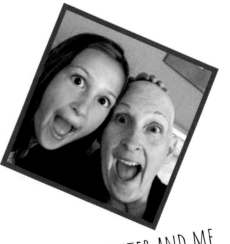

Daughter and me

Sexy bald lady!

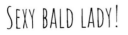

Keep in mind that like cancer, everyone's reaction to chemo is different. I remember a nurse at the infusion center telling me that if I started to feel sick, it would be a couple of days after. Nope! It was almost always 3-5 hours after. I know chemosabes who didn't get sick at all (bastards!). I've done my best to sum up the big parts of the chemo experience. It might be totally different for you. I just hope it doesn't suck too much.

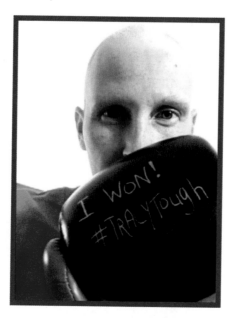

AFTER I GOT THE NEWS THAT I BEAT CANCER. THIS IS MY FAVORITE PICTURE IN THE WHOLE WIDE WORLD BECAUSE I WAS A BADASS.

Prepping for Chemotherapy

You'll hear chemo or chemotherapy referred to as the process, the place, and the medicine. You go to chemo, but you also get chemo. It probably isn't technically right, but it is how people talk.

The place where chemo is done is called an infusion center. These places usually have private "bays" with vinyl hospital style recliners for each patient to chill out in. Where I went, some bays had tv's, some had windows and others were like full on hospital rooms. The one I went to also had a cozy common area with a tv and magazines and a fireplace but it was always empty.

The bays themselves were small, but there was enough room for my husband. He came to every one of my treatments (he is an amazing person). Depending on policies at your hospital, you can probably bring another adult.

Tip: it is a good idea to have a driver or companion (if you take public transportation) the first few times in case you have a reaction or are given medications that make you tired or loopy.

With most types of chemo, you are attached to an IV pole. You are able to get up and walk around or go to the bathroom if you need to. There are types of chemo that do need to be manually fed and you won't be able to move. Your doctor or nurse will let you know and probably have you pee before, if that is the case.

Most people get a port. This is basically a little access panel to your veins to make chemo easier for the nurses. Another option is a pic line. If you get either one of these, you'll have a small procedure to have it put in. From what I'm told, they can be annoying and irritating at first, but you will likely get used to it.

I was an outlier when it came to a port. I never had one and I'm not really sure why my doctor didn't give me one. It was a pain in the ass for the nurses who administered chemo because I had to be stuck every time. In hindsight, I'm glad I didn't have one, but it also may have made the process easier.

You'll likely get an on-body injector for a special shot you might get after each infusion. The shot helps your body make white blood cells so that you can fight any illness that you are exposed to. The on-body injector makes it so that you don't have to go back to the doctor to get a shot the day after your treatment.

On chemo day, make sure you wear something so that there is easy access to your port, pic line, or a vein in your arm. Button up shirts, zip up sweatshirts, a loose tee shirt, or a flannel are always a good bet. Hoodies are the most comfortable thing in the world, but for chemo they don't work.

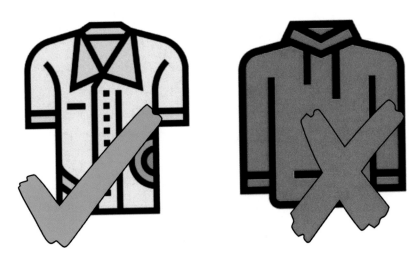

There is a bunch of advice online about what to bring to the infusion center. The first few times, I had a huge tote bag packed. A lot of what is on those lists of what to bring is available at the infusion center. They have mints and gum and blankets and all sorts of stuff. When it came down to it, all I really needed was my phone and a good book if I was in the mood to read. They will likely have a small library at your infusion center, so the book isn't necessary.

A word of warning: chemo is cold! Even if it is 100 degrees outside, you will freeze when that cold poison hits your veins. Be prepared. I highly recommend comfy socks or slippers (they usually have something but they are hospital grade). If you are bald, bring a hat or some type of head covering.

After the first time or two, you'll pretty much know what you need going forward. I definitely over packed.

Stuff the internet tells you to bring to the infusion center:

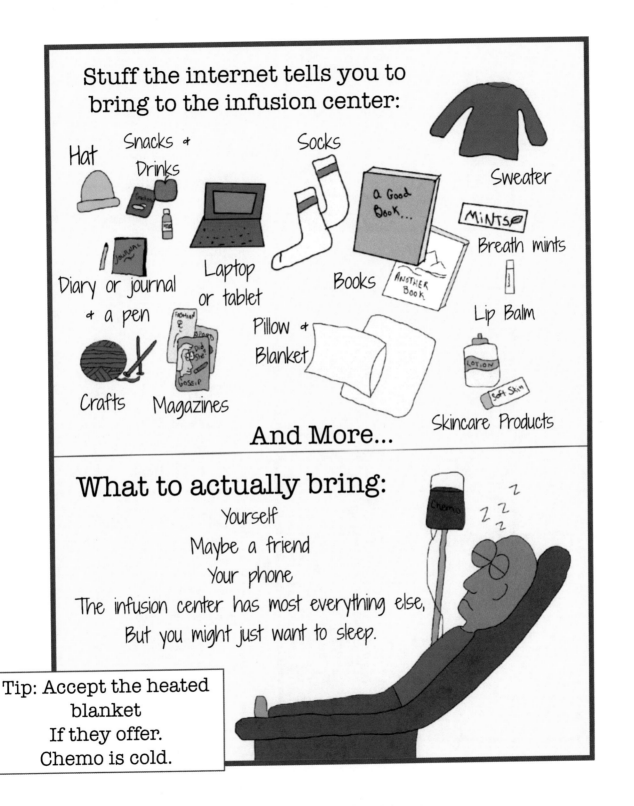

Hat

Snacks & Drinks

Socks

Sweater

A Good Book...

ANOTHER Book

MINTS

Breath mints

Lip Balm

Diary or journal & a pen

Laptop or tablet

Books

LOTION

Soft Skin

Crafts

Magazines

Pillow & Blanket

Skincare Products

And More...

What to actually bring:

Yourself

Maybe a friend

Your phone

The infusion center has most everything else,

But you might just want to sleep.

Chemo

Z Z Z

Tip: Accept the heated blanket
If they offer.
Chemo is cold.

When it is go time, beware of the pre infusion saline flush! You can taste it when it goes into your veins. I'm not sure if the saline flush is really that bad for most people, but for me, the taste triggers bad feelings (PTSD, most likely). I tried Altoids and Jolly Ranchers, but because of the association with that saline taste, I can't stomach them, even years later.

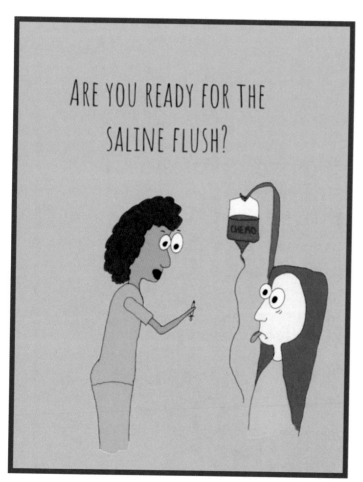

Tip: If the taste is a problem for you, try breathing through your mouth When the nurse starts the flush. You won't taste it as much. See? Mouth breathers aren't so bad after all.

Hair!
Or lack thereof...

The most commonly known side effect of chemotherapy is losing your hair. There are some chemo cocktails that don't cause hair loss and some people don't lose their hair, but for the most part, accept that you're probably gonna be bald. And if you are on the type of chemo that doesn't make you bald, read this stuff, laugh, and be grateful you aren't dealing with it.

The hair doesn't fall out immediately, it usually starts about two weeks after your first treatment. Someone in your life or online will inevitably suggest cold capping. This is basically an ice pack for your head that helps you not lose hair. Everyone I personally know who did it say it isn't worth the trouble. They lost patches of hair anyway and after chemo, their hair came back different, just like everyone who embraced the bald.

Tip: If your hair is longer, cut it short before it starts to fall out. A couple weeks later, shave it before it really starts to go. It comes out in clumps.

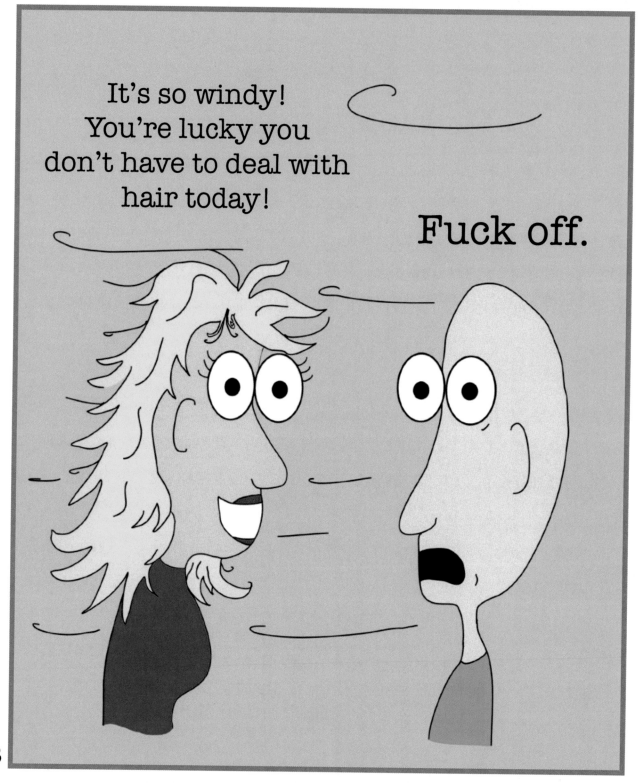

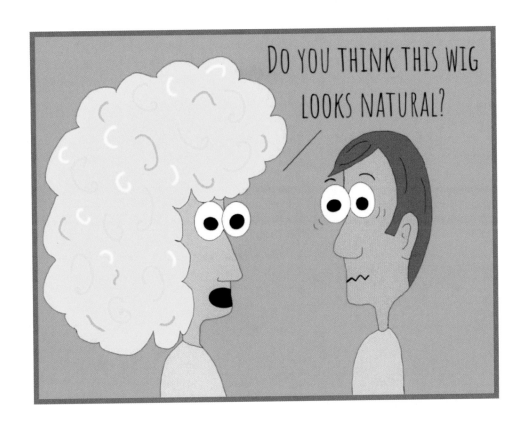

Wigs are an option. But many look fake, no matter how high quality or expensive they are. Do your research if you are going for a natural look. You also have the option of just having fun with them. My favorite wig was bright pink!

Tip: Just be a bald person. It's less stressful once you get used to it. Not too many people will stare, I promise.

Bald is Beautiful!

10 Reasons being bald is actually pretty great

10. Change your hairstyle as often as you want with wigs.

9. People are extra nice and patient with you because you have cancer.

8. Bald is sexy, no matter your gender. See: Dwayne Johnson, Natalie Portman, Patrick Stewart, RuPaul Charles, you.

7. It teaches you self confidence.

6. It feels really good when it is hot outside or if you have hot flashes & night sweats.

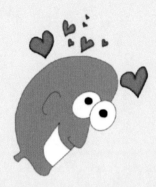

5. So many options for costume parties... Charlie Brown, Mr. Clean, Eleven, a Baby, any ball.

4. You save money on haircare.

3. You can wear cool hats and not look like a douchebag or wannabe fashionista.

2. No Shaving. Anywhere! For months!

1. You can say, "I woke up like this!" And it is true!

Depending on the type of chemo you have, it will probably be two or three weeks after your first infusion before your hair starts going. I got my hair cut short prior to starting chemo- it was a leap of faith because I'd only ever had chin length or long hair because I was convinced I would look bad. Turns out, I love it short (other than sometimes being called "sir").

Shave your head or have a friend do it before things really go south. I knew it was time to shave when I ran my fingers through my hair and it came out between my fingers. I was on the way home from my second chemo, so it was exactly two weeks.

Tip: If you really want to have fun, do your shaving over a few days. Maybe shave your temples at first. Then the next day, have it shaved up the back or carve a design in. Another day, a mohawk. I feel like I missed the boat on this one.

After you've shaved, use duct tape to pull out the stubble, otherwise you'll be shedding tiny hairs all over your pillow. It doesn't hurt and is oddly satisfying to get a nice piece of tape covered in stubble.

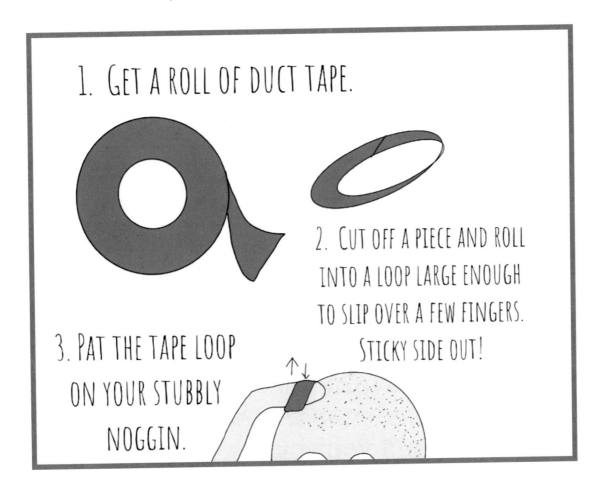

1. GET A ROLL OF DUCT TAPE.

2. CUT OFF A PIECE AND ROLL INTO A LOOP LARGE ENOUGH TO SLIP OVER A FEW FINGERS. STICKY SIDE OUT!

3. PAT THE TAPE LOOP ON YOUR STUBBLY NOGGIN.

You probably are only really concerned with the hair on your head, but your have hair all over your body. I'm stating the obvious here: You will lose all of your hair. <u>ALL OF IT.</u>

Eyebrows, eyelashes, arm hair, leg hair, facial hair, armpit hair, and the hair down there. One of the big "bonuses" of chemo is you get a break from shaving. Yay, I guess.

Regarding pubes... if you don't do a full landscaping job, at some point you'll discover what looks like a squirrel exploded in your underwear.

Tip: For the love of God, if you normally don't wear underwear please do. No one wants to find your pubes all over the place. Keep that shit contained!

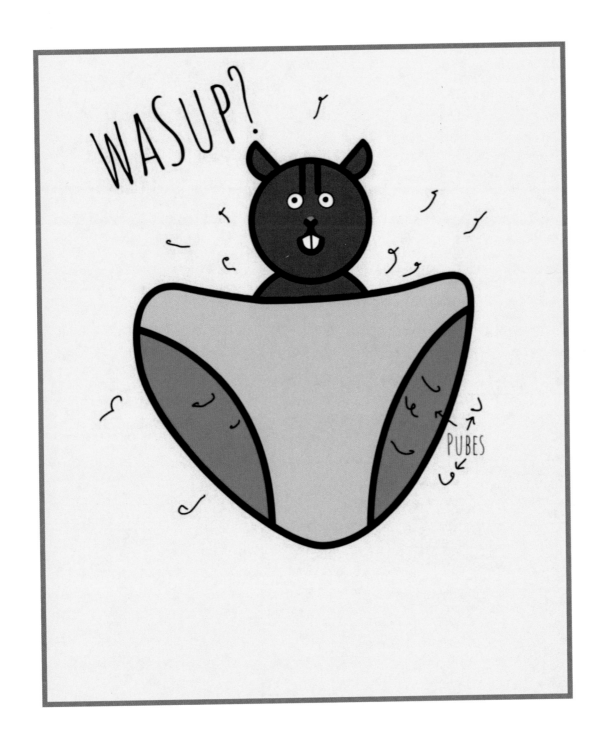

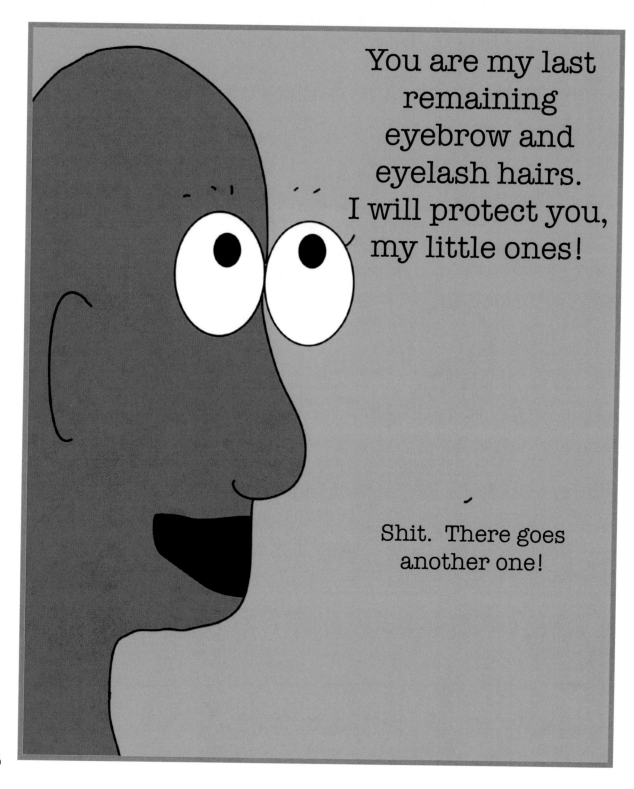

The good news is that for most of us, hair comes back. But there is a chance that your hair won't be what it was pre-chemo. Some people get lucky and end up with better than what they had before. Others, not so much,

My pre chemo hair was full and curly to the point it was out of control. It wasn't "good hair" by any means, but if I took my time it could look nice. After chemo it is baby fine and straight. It is basically like a toddler's hair. I hate it and really miss my curls.

It is common for color to change as well. I know several people, mostly over age 40, who ended up with gray hair. Some people who had gray hair pre chemo get color post chemo. I know a young woman who was blonde grow dark hair after chemo.

I went from brown hair to gray. I am not quite ready to rock my gray, so I color my hair. I don't have issues, even though it is much finer than before. Consult with your stylist on this.

Hair Before Chemo

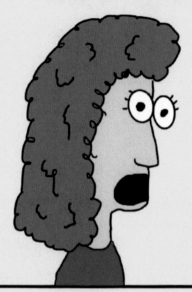

Ugh! I hate my hair! I wish is was straight and this color is so blah!

Hair After Chemo

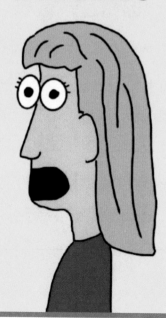

Ugh! I hate my hair! I wish it was curly and this color is so blah!

Other body parts related to hair that can be affected by chemo are your fingernails and toenails. If you're into manicures, pedicures, or wear acrylics, you will be forced to take a break from those things for a bit. You need to avoid things that will potentially cause an infection.

Some people lose their nails completely. Others have issues with color or texture. I got through all of my treatments with no issues whatsoever. But after treatment... my nails grew in brown and lifted a little. They mostly recovered after about a year (but are more brittle than before).

I didn't get a professional mani or pedi until I was long past a risk of infection or having a nail pop off in a nail tech's face. I did at home nail care. I hid the discoloration with polish or nail wraps. My doctor had no issue with this but some doctors might feel differently, so consult accordingly.

This was taken nearly a year after my final chemo. It was just before I cut off my last chemo remnant. As you can see, it was brown and the tip was lifted a bit. It took another year or so for the lifted tip to return to normal.

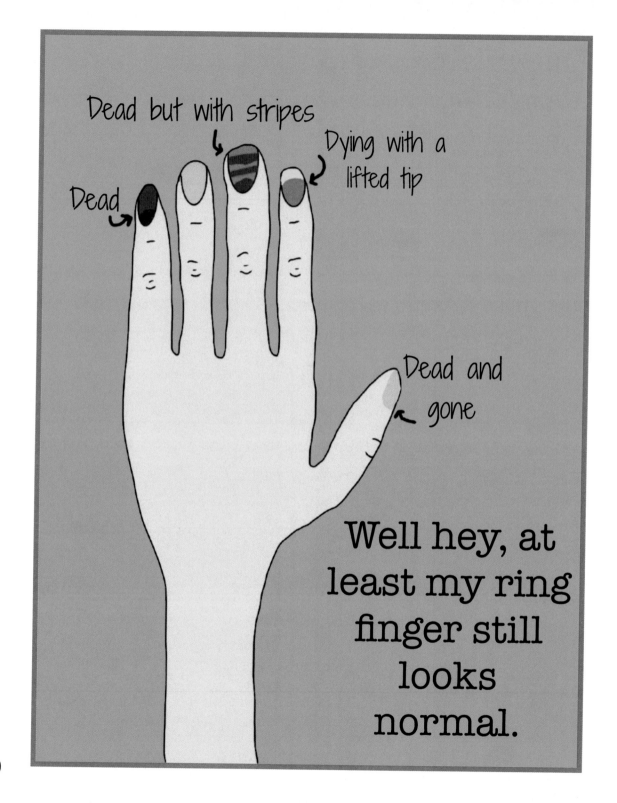

Try to Remember that People Mean Well...

If you think that people piss you off when you are healthy, it is a million times worse when you aren't. You're going to be constantly bombarded with advice whether you want it or not. People might say stupid shit. Everyone wants to help but they don't always go about it in the most sensitive way. Sometimes fellow humans just don't know what to say so they might outright avoid or ignore you. Don't take it personally. Do your best not to throat punch anyone during this rough time in your life.

Tip: People are going to want to help you. Let them! If they want to clean your house or do your dishes, awesome. If they want to bring you food, please oblige. And if they want to give you money, don't be too proud to take it. Accepting money can be a tough thing, but keep in mind that if someone wants to give it to you, they probably have enough to spare. **That is their way of helping**. If you are fortunate enough not to need it, you can always give to charity. Remember to pay it forward when you are healthy, whether it be donating time or money.

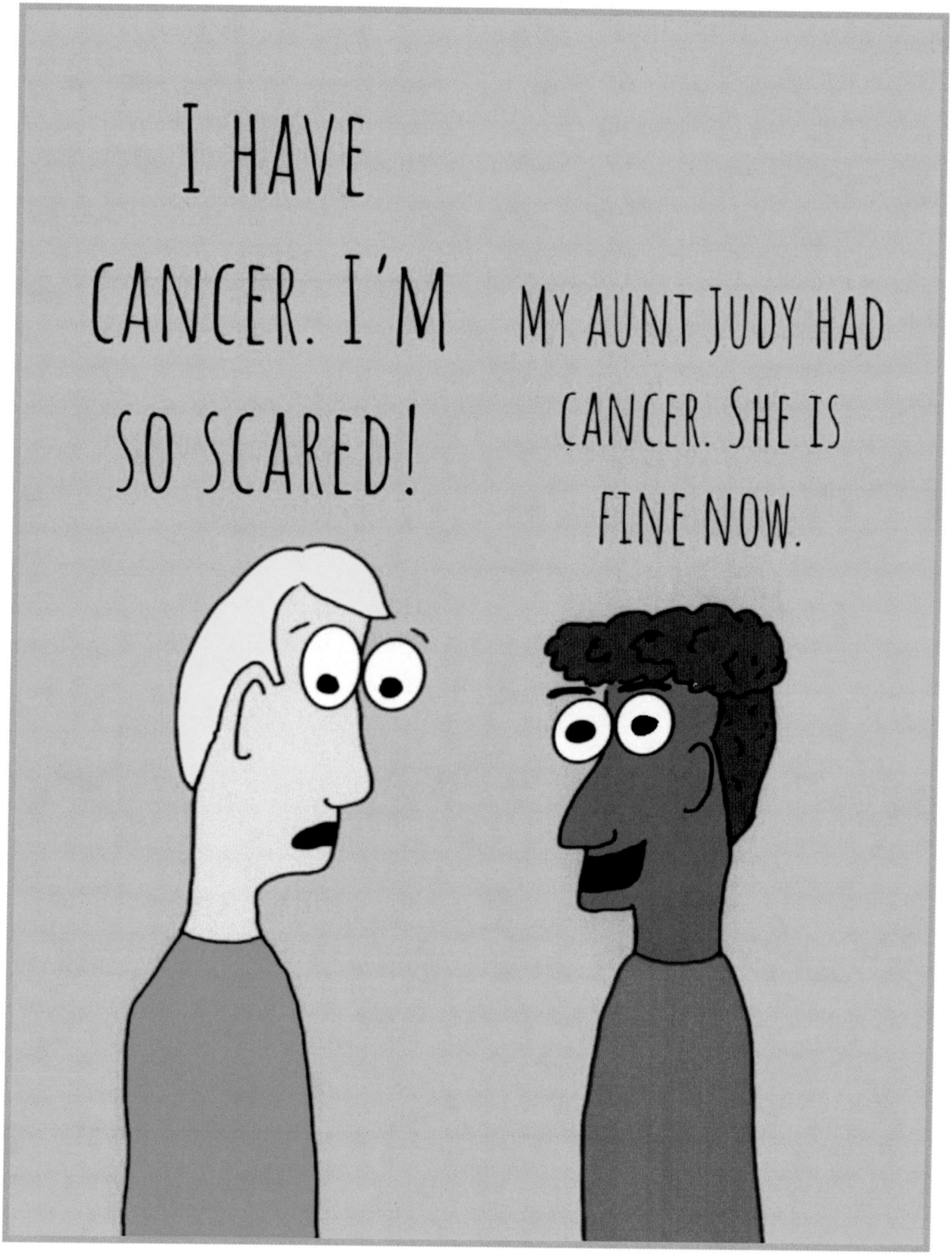

This is YOUR cancer. You get to treat it the way you feel is best for you. You'll get some pretty crazy advice about natural methods for treatment. You're probably going to read up on stuff because chemo really does suck. If you are reading this book, you and your doctor have obviously decided that chemo is the best treatment for you.

Oh, but you'll get advice. People are going to attempt to sell you cures and send you scary statistics about chemo. They're going to tell you that they read about or saw a documentary from a guy who cured his cancer by eating a certain way or taking a certain product. You will get lots of advice, whether you want it or not. I still see people telling cancer patients to try this or that.

Chemo is so bad for you. I heard about some guy who drank vitamin infused llama urine and danced naked in the street twice a week and it cured him. You should Google for ideas on how to cure yourself. Big Pharma doesn't want you to get better. They buy the cures when they get discovered to keep people sick!

Thanks, but my doctor has treated hundreds of patients. I think I'll rely on her.

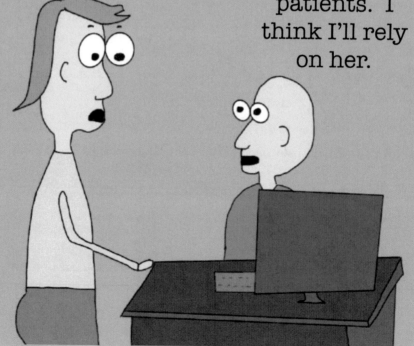

Two things to consider when someone gives you chemo advice:

1. Is the person who is giving the advice a cancer survivor who used this method or did they just read about it, see a video, or hear it through the grapevine?

2. If it is someone who claims to have cured themselves or someone else without chemo, are they trying to sell you something?

If you do want to try miracle oils or pills and alternative cures, just be sure it doesn't interfere with the chemo. I personally had reiki, thanks to a friend who wanted to work with me. It was pretty cool. I also did visualization exercises. And with my doctor's blessing, I took a supplement for neuropathy in my feet that was caused by chemo. Use your best judgement and of course always consult your doctor(s) on this stuff.

I'm secretly hoping that chemo will give me super powers.

Eating

Not gonna lie- I love food. I'm pretty sure I'm addicted to every bad food on the planet. I was prior to cancer and probably more so after. In fact, I ate pretty healthy and worked out when I was diagnosed, so now I just enjoy all the food. Even though I was into fitness and good nutrition at that time in my life, I got sick anyway (no, I don't carry any cancer genes).

One of the many weird chemo side effects is that it affects your sense of taste. It basically kills your taste buds. I could only really taste sweet and spicy. Everything else was bland and gross. I have always been really good about drinking water, but during chemo, I didn't even want it! For some reason, lemonade was really damn good. Instead of drinking regular lemonade, I got True Lemon drink mixes to add to my water. They contain stevia, so it is better than sugar. And you can get them at Walmart or Amazon or pretty much anywhere.

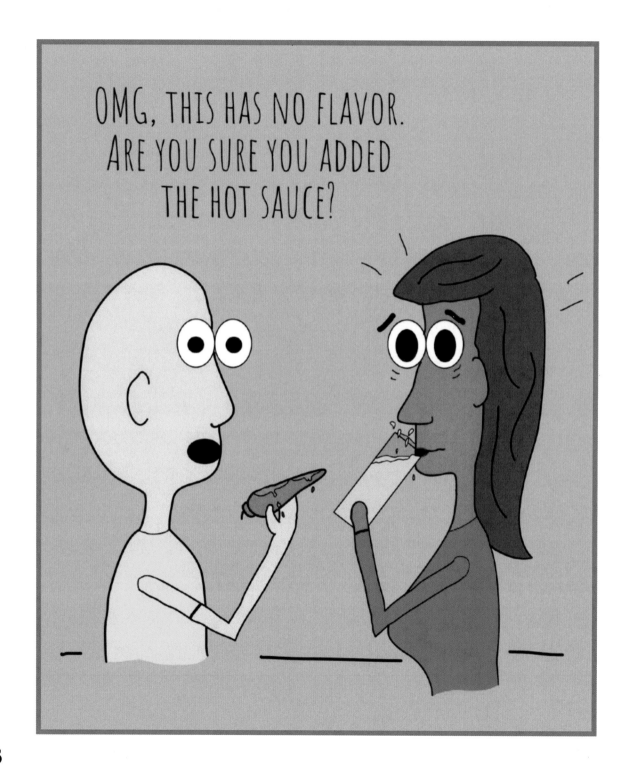

In all honesty, sometimes you just aren't hungry. You know you should eat, but your body is breaking itself down and simultaneously healing, so it really doesn't want food. On top of that, everything tastes weird.

There is one thing that I could stomach during my bad days:

APPLESAUCE

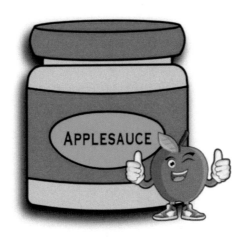

It is sweet (one flavor I could taste), soft, relatively nutritious and since I had chemo during the summer months, I appreciated that it was cold.

Tip: If you've ever been pregnant (sorry guys), your tastes are a bit similar. I had the same issue with not liking water during both of my pregnancies. I preferred lemonade and sucking on ice to get hydration. Other similarities was that minty toothpaste was gross and made me gag.

There was a weird phenomenon in my chemo support group. Anywhere from 3 to 5 days post infusion, everyone seemed to crave greasy, bad food! Cheeseburgers, tacos, fast food, bar food, whatever nasty delicious food is out there- we all seemed to want it. There were even vegetarians in my group who wanted a big 'ol juicy burger. Some people are pretty strict with their diets during chemo and it is totally up to you as to what you want to do- but after 5 days of applesauce, I had the damn burger!

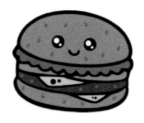

The Nitty Gritty
(and Sometimes Gross)
Reality of Chemo

You know you're probably going to go bald. And you've heard that sometimes people get sick. But this part of the book is the nitty gritty. The stuff that sometimes nobody talks about or when it is, it is talked about in such a politically correct way that it doesn't sound that bad.

You're about to get this information the most direct, blunt, and simple way that you can.

You've been warned.

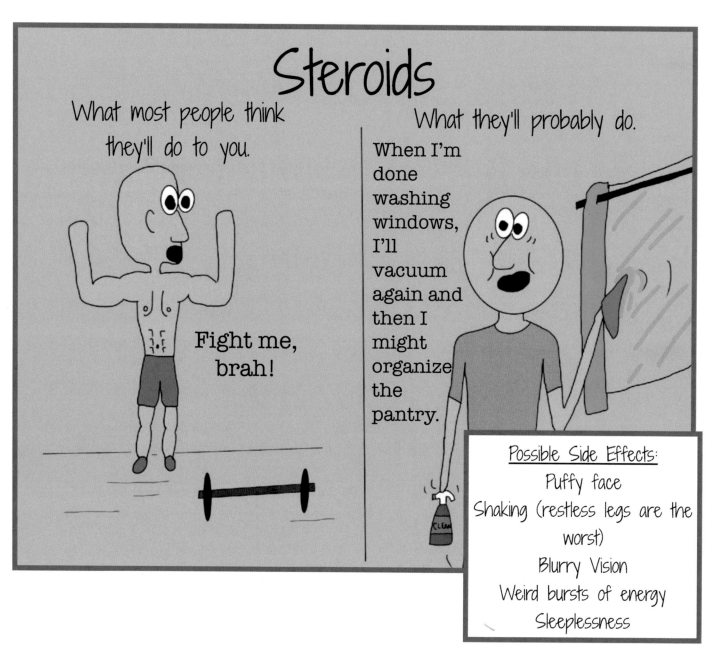

42

Roid Rage & Puking

You are probably going to be prescribed steroids. Why? They reduce inflammation, can help your appetite, keep your energy up, and can also help you feel better.

With roids, you might not get out of bed for days, or you might have more energy than you've ever had in your entire life. It isn't a pleasant energy, more like movement you can't get rid of, but you feel too shitty to exercise. They also make you a little crazy and confused, so try not to make any major life decisions at this time.

Your doctor doesn't want you to puke. They'll give you anti nausea drugs for that purpose. If you do puke more than a couple of times, they will probably want you to call in. I personally did puke way more than they wanted me to and different meds did nothing. It was brutal. My awesome husband called the doctor late at night and ended up going to an overnight pharmacy to get me a new med when the first one didn't work.

But for the record, it sounds like most people are able to control their nausea. I was just unlucky. I have heard that CBD oil can help. At the time of my diagnosis, it was illegal in my state. But for many, I am hearing that it can help.

Tip: Stay ahead of your anti nausea meds. If you miss one or don't take it like clockwork you will pay the price.

As a cancer survivor, the number one question I am asked most by people who are currently in chemo is:

How in the hell do I make this neuropathy go away?

The Mayo Clinic website defines neuropathy as "a result of damage to the nerves outside of the brain and spinal cord (peripheral nerves), often causes weakness, numbness and pain, usually in your hands and feet. It can also affect other areas of your body... Peripheral neuropathy can result from traumatic injuries, infections, metabolic problems, inherited causes and exposure to toxins."

Did you read that? EXPOSURE TO TOXINS. That's us!

Neuropathy feels like burning, tingling, numbness, or pain. It is obviously different for everyone. The closest feeling I can describe is when your foot falls asleep. It doesn't feel "normal" and is annoying. Only with neuropathy, it never stops feeling that way. I always had it worse in my hands and my right foot. I would smack the affected body part against a chair or the table just to feel a different sensation.

Some people lose all feeling with neuropathy. A friend of mine told me a story about how his dad completely lost all feeling in his hands and took a pan out of the oven with no oven mitts. He simply forgot to put them on. He also burnt the shit out of his hands because that is what happens when you have skin.

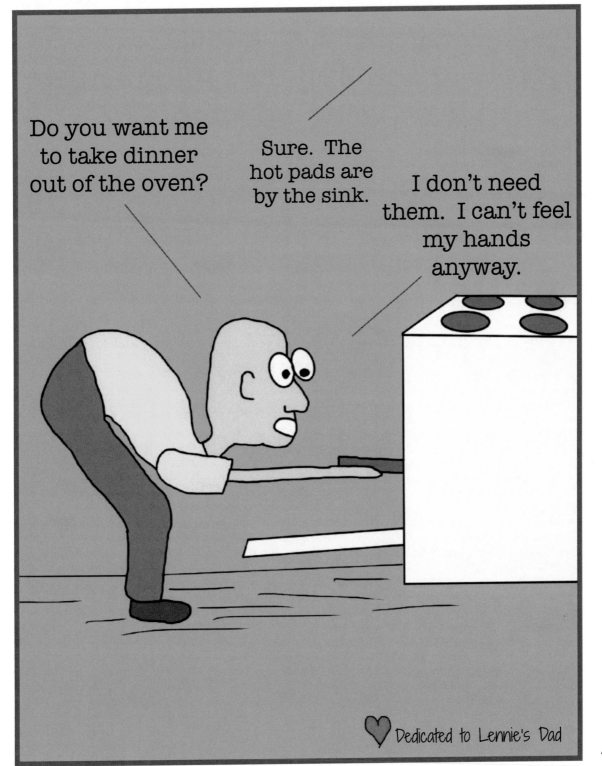

How in the hell do I make this neuropathy go away???

Sadly, for some people, it never goes away. I suppose you get used to it or it becomes the new normal. Mine definitely improved but I still get bouts of it. It tends to flare up in my right foot and right hand with weather changes or stress and is not nearly as intense as it used to be. But for the most part, I don't live with it on a day to day basis.

Let me stress that I AM NOT A DOCTOR, so if you want to try what I did, please talk to yours first. I used a supplement called glutamine. In fact, many doctors recommend it. I used a powdered version that I ordered online and had a scoop of it every day in a drink or in applesauce. I believe there are pills as well.

I believe it helped me, but I know it doesn't work for everyone.

Be a Smart Mouth!

Your mouth is a precious commodity. It feeds you and it creates sound so you can communicate. And when it is "off" you notice. I'm sorry to inform you, but like everything else, chemo will do weird and uncomfortable things to your mouth.

There is a lot of information out there about chemo mouth sores so I won't get into detail. I personally did not experience them, although I did suck on ice in the beginning. I'm not sure if I just got lucky or if the ice helped. It is worth a try, if the ice doesn't bother you.

I did get a gross feeling in my mouth a lot. It was sort of like dry cotton mouth with socks on your teeth. The one thing that helped was a product called Biotene. They make toothpaste and mouthwash. I had both but usually just used the toothpaste. It is "softer" than normal toothpaste. It is hard to describe unless you experience it, but trust me, if you get gross mouth, you'll appreciate this stuff!

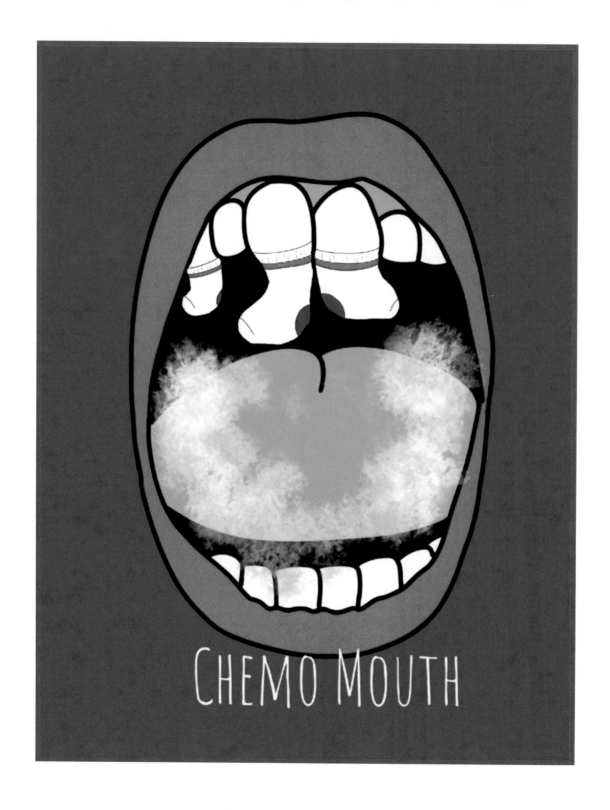

Jeepers, Creepers, I Can't Deal With My Peepers

Something else on your face that can be affected by the poison raging in your system are your eyes. This could be related to the steroids or the chemo itself.

Some people experience an increase in tears and deal with watering eyes. Blurry vision is very common. Sensitivity to light is also normal so make sure you wear sunglasses outdoors (and sometimes indoors). You'll also learn to keep lights low in the house.

Prior to chemo, I really only wore glasses to drive or watch tv. After, I seemed to have developed astigmatism and wear them almost constantly. I'm convinced that it did something to my eyesight. In doing some research for this book, my experience is not uncommon. I also read an account of a woman who's eyes lost pigment and changed from brown to blue!

Tip: Download some podcasts. Watching TV, staring at phone screens, and reading can be uncomfortable.

It Puts the Lotion on it's Skin...

It goes without saying but your skin, the largest organ in your body, will show the affects of chemo. Dry, rough and itchy skin is really common. Don't be afraid to spend money on a good quality lotion. Some people recommend unscented products. If your skin is in really bad shape, try moisturizing with mineral oil or a super thick ointment called Aquaphor.

Sunscreen is a no brainer here... don't go out without it.

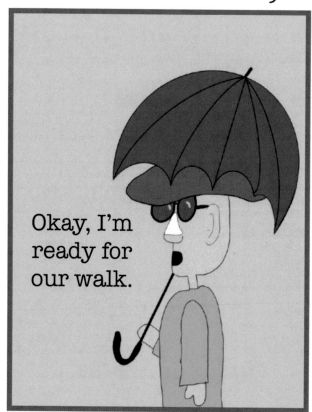

Okay, I'm ready for our walk.

Potty Time

I'm about to talk shit and it won't be pretty.

Chemo potty time is not a pleasant, emptying your bowels experience. Other than the politically correct doctor speak of "you may experience loose bowels or constipation" that is usually about all you hear. I'm about to tell you the ugly truth.

Taking a shit on chemo is excruciating. I became constipated but when it was time to go, everything was dry and painful. I developed hemorrhoids and anal fissures. An anal fissure is a tear in your butthole. Imagine having a torn tater hole and then having to work out a dry, hard turd. Even nuggets were painful.

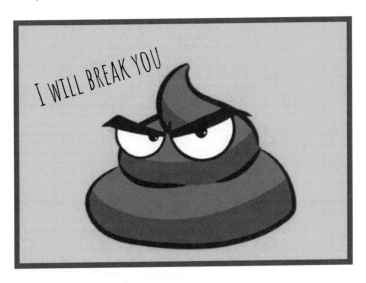

I WILL BREAK YOU

My most traumatic chemo crap was about a week after my first treatment. I was feeling decent enough that I had gone to the gym for a light workout that morning.

I had been constipated, so when the cramps hit, I knew it was time. The pain from the cramps was so intense that I started having hot flashes and sweating. The only thing I wanted to do was get my clothes off. Of course, having been to the gym, I had on a sports bra. I was soaking wet with sweat, in pain, sitting on the toilet trying to shit all while attempting to get a tight sports bra off of a wet body.

I became drenched in sweat to the point that my hair looked like I had just been in the shower (this was before I lost my hair, obviously). I was a woman on a mission and managed to strip all of my clothes off while sitting on the toilet. The cramps would not stop- it was like I was being ripped apart from the inside. I was home alone, which was both a blessing and a curse. No one was there to see me in this state, but no one was there to call for help.

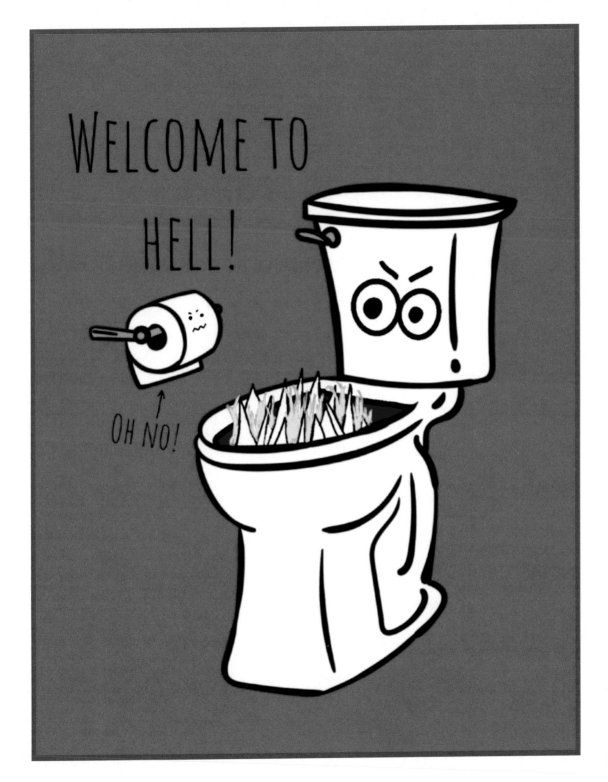

The only way to end the pain was to make the poop come out. The cramps were like labor contractions and that turd was my baby. After some time trying to give birth, I'd take a break and lay on the floor, sweaty and naked. I may have puked a time or two- I don't remember. The pain was bad enough that I debated calling my doctor or even 911. Of course the last thing you want to deal with in a small town is having the volunteer EMT squad, consisting of your kids' friends' parents and gossip hounds to take you to the hospital because you couldn't poop. The thought of that only motivated me more.

After several bouts of stomach cramps and moving myself off and on the toilet in between pushing, I finally pooped. I don't think it was anything special and angels didn't sing, but I had finally completed my mission.

I was so exhausted afterwards that I collapsed on my bed, naked and drenched in sweat. My mom had been staying with us to help me care for the kids and she got home from where ever she had gone. She found me on the bed in that state. It was not a proud moment in my life. A good sleep later and everything was better.

In talking to other chemo survivors I discovered that I was not alone in this horrific experience. I never had another poop like that, thankfully. I do believe that poop may have caused anal fissures and after that, toilet time was painful for weeks. My kids still talk about me screaming in pain whenever I had to take a dump. Aside from the poop, the farts smell lethal.

Tip: I don't want this to happen to another soul, so please, make sure you stay hydrated any way you can. Stool softeners and fiber supplements eventually made a difference as well. Make sure you have something on hand! I also bought a Squatty Potty and I love that damn thing to this day.

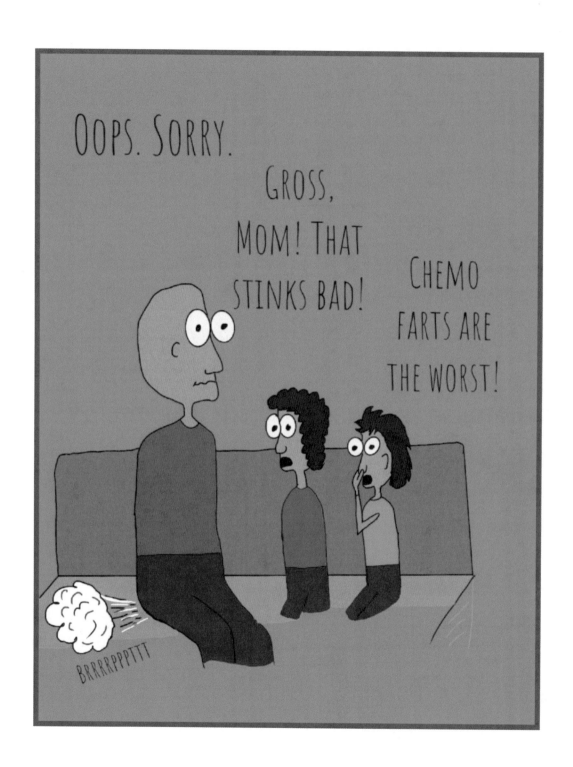

That snot all, folks!

Since we are on the subject of gross things, I want to give you fair warning about one more chemo side effect that nobody really talks about.

Snot.

Remember the part where I said you will lose ALL of your hair? I forgot to mention nose hair. Those little hidden and sometimes annoying but forgotten about hairs actually have a job when it comes to your biology. They slow down the flow of mucous. And holy shit, when you don't have nose hair, you understand how important it is.

I don't know if chemo changes the consistency of your snot or if it is always like water and the hair stops the constant flow. But please, never leave the house without tissues or a handkerchief. Your nose will drip all the time, even if it is summer.

> Tip: Have tissues stashed everywhere! Put a box in every room in your house, in your car, in your office, and definitely in your pocket.

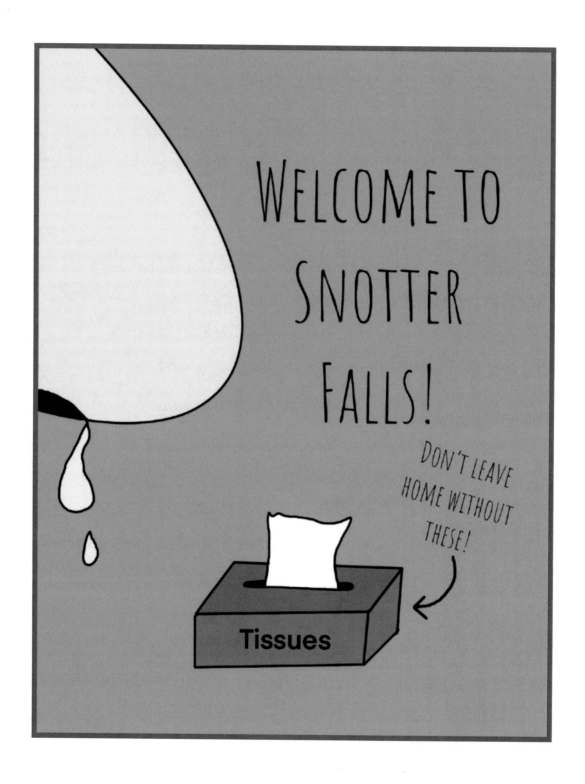

60

The Small Silver Linings

Chemotherapy is horrible. The reason for having it is even worse. But ultimately it can save your life, so you have faith in modern medicine and you deal with the shit in the hopes you get to stay on this spinning rock hurling through space for years to come.

There are some very, very minor benefits though. One is that your morning routine goes fast because you don't have hair to wash in the shower. So, you can sleep in for a bit!

I had chemo during the summer and both of my kids play ball. Apparently the bugs were pretty bad that year, but they didn't touch me. My guess is that the bugs knew I was toxic.

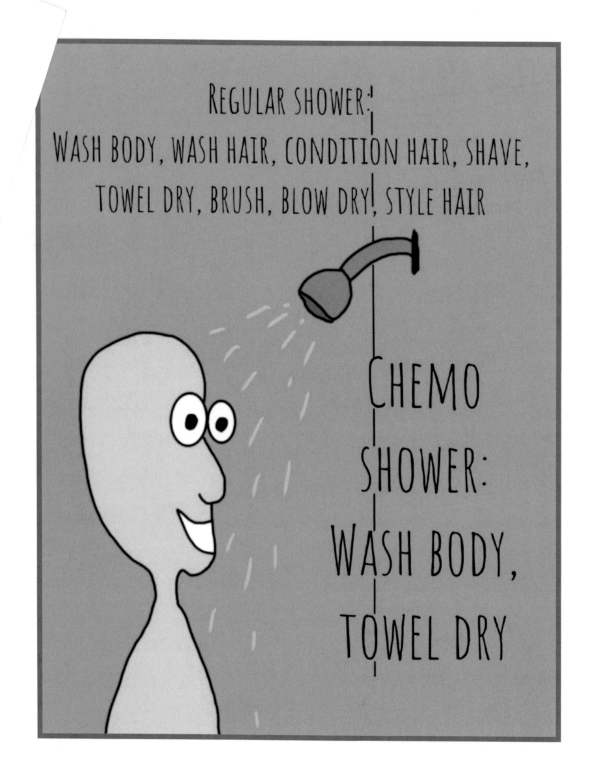

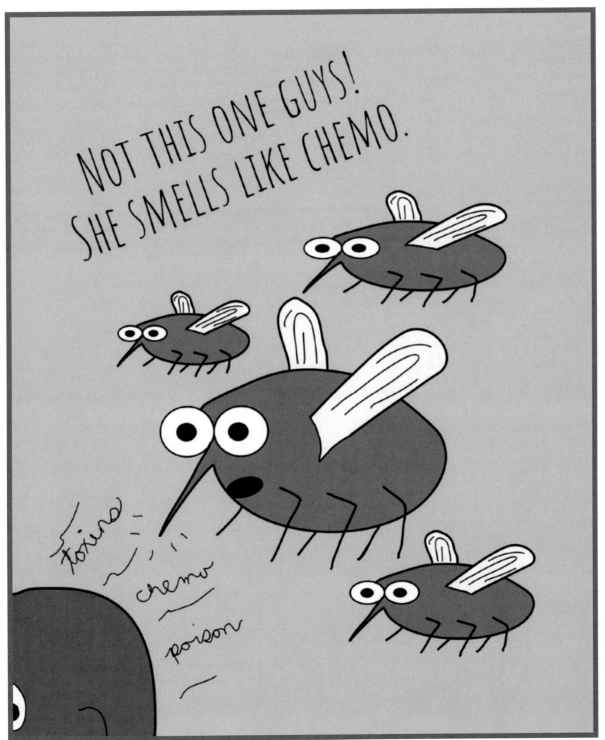

Probably the most impactful silver lining after going through chemo is the perspective you gain. You will be forever changed.

You no longer take the little things for granted. You might be more cautious- or maybe you decide to take more risks. You have empathy in situations that you maybe didn't understand before. You truly get that life is short. And, you know that you are strong and you are a bad ass.

I am one of the lucky ones. I know this every day that I live and breathe. If you end up like me, please make it your mission to be a better person, help others by sharing your experience, be kind. If your battle is one that you will ultimately lose, please know that you are loved and that people who you don't even know will grieve for you. That is part of being a survivor- we truly hurt when one of our own doesn't make it.

But we are all here at this moment. Go out there, kick ass, and get through chemo with a smile on your face. Hopefully this stupid book has helped. Also, fuck cancer.

I hope that someday Cancer is just a zodiac sign.

Helpful Items to Have While You are on Chemo

These are things mentioned in this book so that you have a list in one place

- True Lemon drink mixes
- Applesauce
- Warm fuzzy socks
- Bandanas or soft caps
- Duct Tape
- Glutamine (I used NOW brand in powder form)
- Fiber supplement
- Stool softeners
- Biotene Toothpaste and Mouthwash
- Tissues
- Sunglasses
- A good quality lotion: Aveno, Nutragena, or your usual lotion
- Sunscreen
- Squatty Potty
- Don't forget to download some podcasts!